Understanding Cancer of the Ovary

Published by BACUP
121/123 Charterhouse Street, London, EC1M 6AA
Administration: 01 608 1785
Cancer Information Service: 01 608 1661 (6 lines)

Charity Registration No. 290526

© BACUP, 1987
All rights reserved. No part of this publication may be reproduced or transmitted, in any form or by any means, electronic or mechanical, including photocopying, recording or any information storage and retrieval system, without permission in writing from BACUP.

The publishers gratefully acknowledge the support of Bristol Myers Oncology in the production of this booklet.

BACUP stands for the British Association of Cancer United Patients. It was founded in 1984 by Dr Vicky Clement-Jones, following her own experiences with ovarian cancer, and offers information, advice and emotional support to cancer patients and their families and friends.

BACUP produces a range of publications on the main types of cancer, their treatments, and different ways of living and coping with cancer. We also produce a newspaper, *BACUP News*, which is published three times a year.

BACUP's success depends largely on the feedback we receive from users of the service. We would like to thank all those people, particularly patients and their families, whose valuable comments and advice have made this booklet possible.

Editor: Dr Maurice Slevin, MD, MRCP

Deputy Editor: Sally Watts, SRN

Publications Consultant: Elizabeth Sturgeon

Cover illustration by Malcolm Harvey Young

ISBN 1-870403-07-X

Contents

Introduction	2
What Is Cancer?	3
The Ovaries	4
What Causes Cancer of the Ovary?	5
What Are the Symptoms of Cancer of the Ovary?	5
How Does the Doctor Make the Diagnosis?	6
What Types of Treatment Are Used?	11
Surgery	11
After Your Operation	12
Will the Operation Affect My Sex Life?	14
Chemotherapy	15
Side Effects	15
Radiotherapy	17
Planning Your Treatment	17
Side Effects	18
Your Feelings	19
Learning to Cope	22
Who and What to Tell	23
Talking to Children	24
What You Can Do	25
Practical and Positive Tasks	25
Understanding Your Illness	26
Who Can Help?	27
Sick Pay and Benefits	28
BACUP's Cancer Information Service	28
Other Useful Organisations	29
Recommended Reading List	31
Publications Available From BACUP	32

Introduction

This information booklet has been written to help you understand more about cancer of the ovary. We hope it answers some of the questions you may have about its diagnosis and treatment.

We can't advise you about the best treatment for yourself because this information can only come from your own doctor, who is familiar with your full medical history.

At the end of this booklet you will find a list of other BACUP publications, some useful addresses and recommended books. If, after reading this booklet, you think it has helped you, do pass it on to any of your family and friends who might find it interesting. They too may want to be informed so they can help you cope with any problems you may have.

What Is Cancer?

The organs and tissues of the body are made up of tiny building blocks called cells. Cancer is a disease of these cells. Cells in different parts of the body may look and work differently but they repair and reproduce themselves in the same way. Normally, this division of cells takes place in an orderly and controlled manner, but if for some reason this process gets out of control, the cells will continue to divide, developing into a lump which is called a tumour. Tumours can either be benign or malignant.

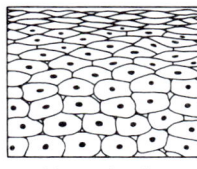 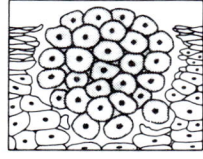

Normal cells **Cells forming a tumour**

In a benign tumour the cells do not spread to other parts of the body and so are not cancerous. However, if they continue to grow at the original site they may cause a problem by pressing on the surrounding organs.

A malignant tumour is made up of cancer cells which have the ability to spread beyond the original site, and if left untreated may invade and destroy surrounding tissues. Sometimes cells break away from the original (primary) cancer and spread to other organs in the body via the bloodstream or lymphatic system. When these cells reach a new site they may go on dividing and form a new tumour, often referred to as a 'secondary' or a 'metastasis'.

Doctors can tell whether a tumour is benign or malignant by examining a small sample of cells (a biopsy) under a microscope.

It is important to realise that cancer is not one disease with a single cause and a single type of treatment. There are more than 200 different kinds of cancer, each with its own name and treatment.

The Ovaries

The ovaries are two small, oval-shaped organs which are part of the female reproductive system. Each month, in women of reproductive age, an egg leaves one of the ovaries and passes down the fallopian tube to the womb (uterus). If the egg is not fertilised by a male sperm it passes out of the womb and is shed, along with the lining of the womb, as part of the monthly cycle or period.

The ovaries also produce the female sex hormones, oestrogen and progesterone. As a woman nears the 'change of life' or menopause she makes less of these hormones and her periods gradually stop.

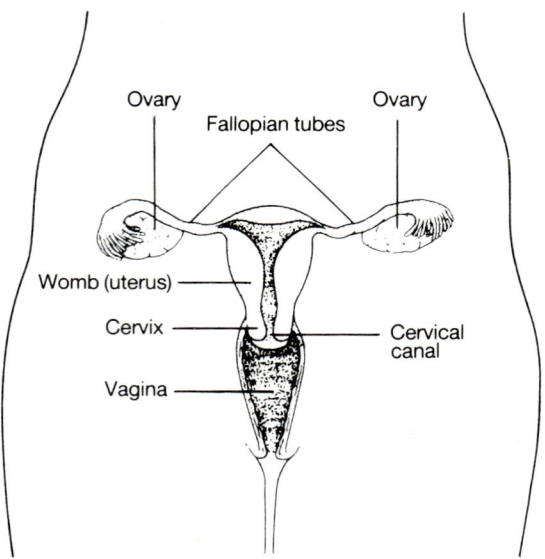

Diagram to show the position of the ovaries

What Causes Cancer of the Ovary?

The cause of cancer of the ovary is unknown. However, it is more common in women who have not had children.

There is strong evidence to suggest that women who are taking the contraceptive pill are less likely to develop this type of cancer.

What Are the Symptoms of Cancer of the Ovary?

Most women with cancer of the ovary don't have any symptoms for a long time. When they do appear they may include any of the following.

Vague indigestion, nausea and a bloated feeling
Swelling in the abdomen — this may be due to a build up of fluid known as ascites
Loss of appetite
Persistent constipation or diarrhoea
Abnormal vaginal bleeding, although this is very rare

If you do have any of the above symptoms you must have them checked by your doctor, but remember, they are common to many other conditions and most women with these symptoms will not have cancer.

How Does the Doctor Make the Diagnosis?

Usually you begin by seeing your family doctor (General Practitioner) who will examine you and arrange for you to have any further tests or X-rays that may be necessary. Your GP may need to refer you to the hospital for these tests and for specialist advice and treatment.

At the hospital the doctor will take your full medical history before doing a physical examination. This will include an internal (vaginal) examination to check for any lumps or swellings. Sometimes your doctor may also want to do an examination of your back passage.

Your doctor may also arrange for you to have a blood test and chest X-ray taken to check your general health.

There are several tests which are used to diagnose cancer of the ovary. They will also show whether or not the disease has spread to other parts of the body. Your doctor may arrange for you to have any of the following tests.

Ultrasound Scan
In this test, sound waves are used to make up a picture of the inside of the abdomen, the liver and the pelvis. It will be done in the hospital scanning department.

Before your test you will be asked to drink plenty of fluids so that your bladder is full and a clear picture can be seen. Once you are lying comfortably on your back a gel is spread over your abdomen. A small probe, like a microphone, which produces sound waves, is then passed over the area. The echoes are converted into a picture by using a computer.

Ultrasound can be used to check for any enlargement or abnormalities of the ovaries which may indicate a cyst or tumour. It is also used to measure the size and position of a cancer.

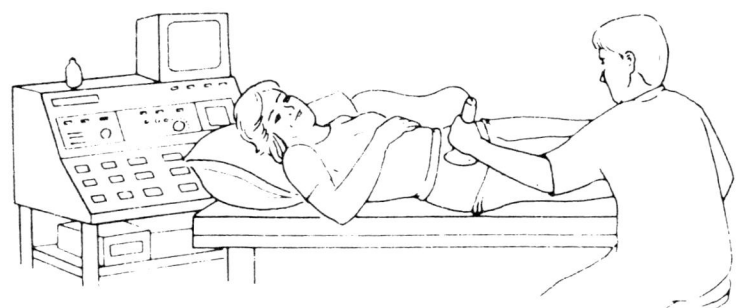

CT (CAT) Scan

A CT scan is a type of X-ray. A number of pictures are taken and fed into a computer to form a detailed picture of the inside of the abdomen, the liver and pelvis. The scan can show the size and position of a cancer.

On the day of your scan you will be asked not to eat or drink anything for at least four hours before your appointment. You will then be given a special liquid, which shows up on X-ray, to drink a few hours before your scan and again in the X-ray department. Just before the scan a similar liquid is passed into your back passage through a small tube and a tampon is put into your vagina. This ensures that a clear picture is obtained.

Once you are lying comfortably on the couch the scan is taken. The scan itself is painless but it will mean lying still for about 30-40 minutes.

Most people are able to go home as soon as their scan is over.

Barium Enema

This is a special X-ray of the bowel. It will be done in the hospital X-ray department.

For the test it is important that the bowel is empty so that a clear picture can be seen. On the day before your test you will be asked to take a laxative and to drink plenty of fluids. On the morning of your enema you should not have anything to eat or drink. This preparation may vary slightly from hospital to hospital but you will be given an instruction sheet to follow.

Just before the test, to make sure that the bowel is completely clear, you may be given a bowel wash-out. For this the nurse will ask you to lie on your side while she gently passes a small tube into your back passage. Water is then passed through the tube and you will be asked to hold this for a few minutes before you go to the toilet.

For the enema a mixture of barium, which shows up on the X-ray, and air is passed into the back passage in the same way as the bowel wash-out so that a clearer picture can be seen. It is important to keep the mixture in the bowel until all the X-rays have been taken. The doctor can then watch the passage of the barium through the bowel on an X-ray screen and any abnormal areas can be seen.

The test can be uncomfortable and tiring and, therefore, it is a good idea to arrange for someone to travel home with you if possible.

For a couple of days after your enema you may notice that your stools are white. This is the barium being removed from the body and is quite normal. The barium can cause constipation and you may need to take a mild laxative for a couple of days after your test.

Intravenous Urogram

This test is also known as an IVU or IVP, and it shows up any abnormalities in the kidneys or urinary system. It will be done in the X-ray department and takes about an hour.

A dye is injected into a vein, usually in the arm, and goes via the bloodstream to the kidneys. The doctor can watch the passage of the dye on an X-ray screen and pick up any abnormalities.

Sometimes the dye can make you feel hot and flushed for a few minutes but this feeling gradually disappears. You should be able to go home as soon as the test is over.

Lymphangiogram (Lymphogram)

This test is done to check for any abnormalities of the lymph nodes in the abdomen and pelvis. It is done in the hospital X-ray department and takes about two to three hours. You may have to go back to the hospital the next day for further X-rays and an IVU.

For the test an oily substance and a dye, which shows up on X-ray, are injected into each foot and pass through the lymphatic vessels to the lymph nodes in the abdomen and pelvis. The doctor can then see on the X-ray the progress of these substances through the vessels and pick up any abnormalities.

The dye that is used in a lymphangiogram can give your skin a green appearance and you may notice that your urine is a bluey-green colour. This is nothing to worry about and usually disappears within 48 hours.

In many hospitals the lymphangiogram has now been replaced by the CAT Scan.

Abdominal Fluid Aspiration

If there has been a build up of fluid in the abdomen a sample can be taken to check for any cancer cells. The doctor will use a local anaesthetic to numb the area before passing a small needle through the skin. Some fluid is drawn off into a syringe and examined under a microscope.

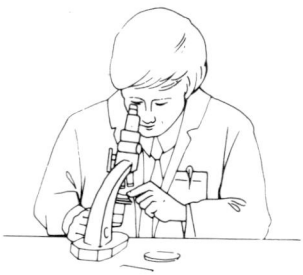

Laparoscopy

This is a small operation which allows the doctor to look at the ovaries and the surrounding area. It is done under a general anaesthetic and will mean a short stay in hospital.

While you are under anaesthetic the doctor makes a small cut in the lower abdomen and carefully inserts a thin, mini-telescope (laparoscope). By looking through the laparoscope the doctor can look at the ovaries and take a small sample of tissue (biopsy) for examination under a microscope.

During the operation, air is passed into the abdominal cavity and this can cause uncomfortable wind pains for a couple of days. The pain is often eased by walking about or by taking sips of peppermint water.

After a laparoscopy you will have one or two stitches in place in your lower abdomen. You should be able to get up as soon as the effects of the anaesthetic have worn off.

It will probably take several days for the results of your tests to be ready and a follow-up appointment will be arranged for you before you go home. Obviously this waiting period is an anxious time for you and it may help you to talk things over with a close friend or relative.

What Types of Treatment Are Used?

Surgery, chemotherapy and radiotherapy may be used alone, or together, to treat cancer of the ovary. Your doctor will plan your treatment by taking into consideration a number of factors including your age, general health, the type and size of the tumour, what it looks like under the microscope and whether it has spread beyond the ovary.

You may find that other women at the hospital are having different treatment from yourself. This will often be because their illness takes a different form, therefore they have different needs. It may also be because doctors take different views about treatment. If you have any questions about your own treatment don't be afraid to ask your doctor or the ward sister. It often helps to make a list of questions for your doctor and to take a close friend or relative with you.

Some women find it reassuring to have another medical opinion to help them decide about their treatment. Most doctors will be pleased to refer you to another specialist for a second opinion if you feel this will be helpful.

Surgery

Your doctor will discuss with you the most appropriate type of surgery, dependent on the type, size and spread of the cancer. Sometimes this information only becomes available during the operation itself and, therefore, it is important to discuss all the possible options with your doctor beforehand. Remember, no operation or procedure will be done without your consent.

Surgery is normally the first treatment for cancer of the ovary. It is usually necessary to remove both ovaries, the fallopian tubes and the womb (hysterectomy). The surgeon may take samples from other tissues, such as the lymph glands to see if the cancer has spread.

If the cancer has already spread to the bowel a small piece of bowel may be removed and the two ends rejoined.

After Your Operation

After your operation you will be encouraged to start moving about as soon as possible. This is an essential part of your recovery and even if you have to stay in bed it is important to keep up regular leg movements and deep breathing exercises.

An intravenous infusion (drip) will be used to replace the body's fluids until you are able to eat and drink again. After an anaesthetic the movement of the gut slows down so it is important that you don't start drinking until it has returned to normal, usually after a few days.

Sometimes a small tube or catheter is put into the bladder and your urine is drained into a collecting bag. You may also have a drainage tube in place from your wound to stop any excess fluid collecting. This is usually removed within 48 hours.

It is quite normal to have some pain or discomfort for a few days but there are several different types of pain-killing drugs which are very effective. If you continue to have pain it is important to let the doctor or ward sister know as soon as possible so that your drugs can be changed.

Most women are able to go home about eight to ten days after their operation, once the stitches or clips have been removed. If you think you might have problems when you go home, for example, if you live alone or have several flights of stairs to climb, let the ward sister or social worker know when you are admitted to the ward so that help can be arranged.

As well as being able to offer practical advice, many social workers are also trained counsellors who can offer valuable support to you and your family, both in hospital and at home. If you would like to talk to a social worker ask your doctor or ward sister to arrange it for you.

Strenuous physical activity or heavy lifting should be avoided for at least three months. Some women also find it uncomfortable to drive for a few weeks after their operation so it may be a good idea to wait a while before you start driving again.

Before you leave hospital you will be given an appointment to attend an Out-Patient clinic for your post-operative check up. This is a good time to discuss any problems you may have after your operation.

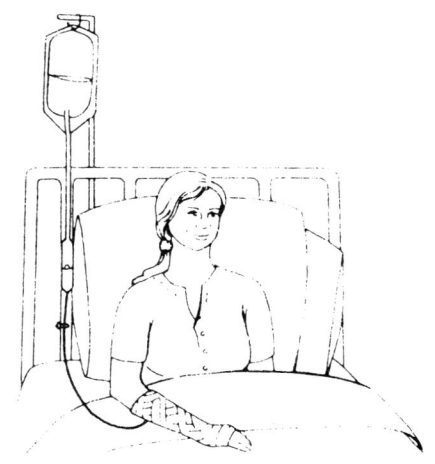

Will the Operation Affect My Sex Life?

One of the common questions which women ask after a hysterectomy is whether the operation will affect their sex life. To allow the wound to heal properly most women are advised to wait at least six weeks after their operation before having sexual intercourse. Many women have no problem resuming a sexual relationship after this time, while others need more time to sort out their emotions.

After a hysterectomy, younger women in particular, often find it difficult to come to terms with the fact they they can no longer have children. They may also be worried that they have lost a part of their female identity. These are very natural, understandable emotions to be experiencing at this time. It can be helpful to discuss any fears or worries with a sympathetic friend or a trained counsellor.

Occasionally there may be a physical reason why a woman is reluctant to have intercourse. For younger women who are still having periods, the removal of the ovaries will bring on an early menopause. The physical effects of this may be hot flushes, dry skin, a dryness of the vagina, which can make sexual intercourse uncomfortable, and a decrease in sexual desire. However, most of these effects can be prevented or reversed by replacing the hormones with tablets or creams. Often a simple lubricant like KY jelly, which can be bought at most chemists, is all that is needed to ease discomfort during intercourse.

One common fear is that cancer can be passed on to your partner during intercourse. This is not true and it is perfectly safe for you to resume a sexual relationship.

Chemotherapy

Chemotherapy is the use of special anti-cancer (cytotoxic) drugs to destroy cancer cells. They work by disrupting the growth of cancer cells.

The drugs are sometimes given orally or, more usually, intravenously (by injection into a vein). Chemotherapy is given as a course of treatment, usually lasting a few days. This is followed by a rest period of a few weeks which allows your body to recover from any side effects of the treatment. The number of courses you have will depend on the type of cancer you have and how well it is responding to the drugs.

Chemotherapy can sometimes be given to you as an out-patient but it will often mean spending a few days in hospital.

Side Effects

While the drugs are acting on the cancer cells in your body they may also reduce temporarily the number of normal cells in your blood. When these cells are reduced you are more likely to get an infection and you may tire easily. During chemotherapy your blood will be tested regularly and, if necessary, you will be given a blood transfusion or antibiotics to treat any infection.

Other side effects may include nausea, vomiting and diarrhoea and sometimes hair loss. Some drugs also make your mouth sore and cause small mouth ulcers. Regular mouthwashes are important and the nurse will show you how to do these properly. If you don't feel like eating you can replace your meals with nutritious high calorie drinks. There are also medicines available from your doctor which stop you feeling sick (anti-emetics).

Although they may be hard to bear at the time, these side effects do disappear once your treatment is over and if you do lose your hair it will grow back surprisingly quickly. Many women cover up their hair loss by wearing wigs, hats or scarves. Most patients are entitled to a free wig from the National Health Service and your doctor or ward sister will be able to arrange this for you.

Not all drugs cause the same side effects and some women have no side effects at all. Your doctor will tell you what problems, if any, to expect from your treatment.

Chemotherapy affects people in different ways. Many are able to lead a normal life during their treatment while others find that they become very tired and have to take things more slowly. Just do as much as you feel like and try not to overdo it.

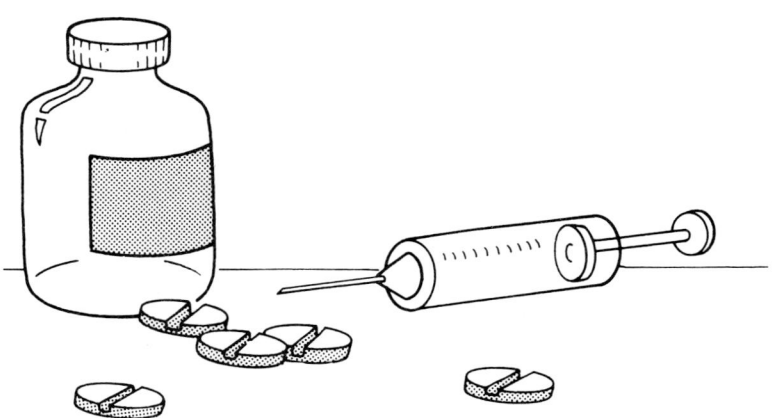

Radiotherapy

Radiotherapy treats cancer by using high energy rays which destroy the cancer cells, while doing as little harm as possible to normal cells.

The treatment is given in the hospital radiotherapy department and the course is usually in five sessions from Monday to Friday, with a rest at the weekend. The length of your treatment will depend upon the type and size of the cancer.

Planning Your Treatment

To ensure that you receive maximum benefit from your radiotherapy it has to be carefully planned. On your first few visits to the radiotherapy department you will be asked to lie under a large machine called a simulator which takes X-rays of the area to be treated. Before the X-rays are taken a tampon is put into your vagina and a liquid, which shows up on X-ray is passed into the back passage. These preparations are done to ensure that the clearest possible pictures are taken. Treatment planning is a very important part of radiotherapy and it may take several visits before the radiotherapist, the doctor who plans your treatment, is satisfied with the result.

Marks will be drawn on your skin to show the radiographer, who gives you your treatment, the exact place for the rays to be directed. During your course of treatment this area should be kept as dry as possible to prevent the skin becoming red and sore.

Before radiotherapy is given the radiographer will position you carefully on the couch and make sure you are comfortable. During your treatment, which only takes a few minutes, you will be left alone in the room but you will be able to talk to the radiographer who will be watching you from an adjoining room.

Radiotherapy is not painful but you do have to lie still for a few minutes while your treatment is being given.

Side Effects

Radiotherapy to the abdomen and pelvic area can cause side effects such as nausea, tiredness, diarrhoea and a burning sensation when passing urine. Many of these side effects can be treated successfully with drugs, so it is important to let your doctor know if you are having any problems. Any side effects will gradually disappear once your course of treatment is over.

While you are having radiotherapy it is important to drink plenty of fluids and maintain a healthy diet. If you don't feel like eating you could try supplementing your meals with high calorie drinks, which are available at most chemists. During your treatment you should try and get as much rest as you can, especially if you have to travel a long way each day.

Radiotherapy does not make you radioactive and it is perfectly safe for you to be with other people, including children throughout your treatment.

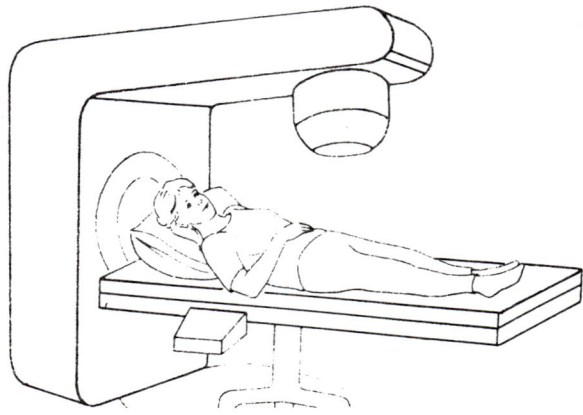

For more information about these treatments and coping with hair loss, see our list of BACUP publications at the end of this booklet.

Your Feelings

Most people are quite overwhelmed when they learn they have cancer. A number of feelings come pouring in which can be muddled and change quickly. Reactions differ from one person to another and this is quite normal. There is no right or wrong way to feel. These feelings are part of the process that people go through in trying to come to terms with their illness. Husbands, friends and family members frequently need as much support and guidance in coping with their feelings as you do.

Shock

'I can't believe it'. 'It can't be true'.

This is often the immediate reaction when someone is told they have cancer. You may feel numb, unable to believe what is happening or to express any emotion. You may find that you can only take in a small amount of information, and find yourself asking the same questions over and over again. This need for repetition is a common reaction to shock.

Denial

'There's nothing wrong with me'. 'I haven't got cancer'.

For many people, not wanting to know is their way of coping with a frightening situation. At this time you may not want to hear any more information. Family members may also react in this way, and sometimes appear to ignore your feelings, 'Don't be silly, it's nothing to worry about'. Being given the opportunity to talk about these feelings can in itself be useful.

Anger

'Why me?' 'This should never have happened'.

Anger can hide other feelings such as fear or sadness. You may be feeling angry, impatient or irritated with those who are closest to you or with the doctors and nurses who are caring for you; perhaps even with God. This is a normal reaction and is a sign of how upset you are about your illness. People around you should not see this as a personal attack against them. If you, or your family, are finding it difficult to cope with these feelings it may be helpful to talk to someone who is less involved in your illness. The nurses at BACUP will be happy to talk to you and offer help and advice with any problems that you may have, either by 'phone or in writing.

Blame and Guilt

'If I hadn't ... this would never have happened'. 'It's my own fault'.

Sometimes people blame themselves or other people for their illness. This may be because we often feel better if we know why something has happened, but since doctors rarely know what has caused an individual cancer, there's no reason for you to blame yourself.

Resentment

'It's all right for you, you haven't got to put up with this'.

This is a nagging, dragging feeling that makes you miserable because you have cancer rather than someone else. Relatives sometimes resent the changes that the patient's illness has made to their life. It may be helpful to bring feelings of resentment out into the open, otherwise they can make everyone feel angry and guilty.

Fear and Uncertainty

'Will the cancer come back?' 'Will the treatment work?'

Cancer is a frightening word surrounded by fears, myths and silence. Fears and fantasies are often worse than the reality. Fear of the unknown can be terrifying so acquiring some knowledge about your illness can often help to lessen this fear. You may be frightened about the future and whether the cancer will come back. Sometimes these fears may emerge as frightening dreams.

Another common fear is that cancer always causes pain. Many patients with cancer experience little or no pain but for those who do, there are many modern pain-relieving drugs which are very successful in keeping it under control.

Withdrawal and Isolation

'Please leave me alone'.

There may be times during your illness when you want to be alone to sort out your thoughts and emotions. This may be upsetting for your family and friends who may want to share this difficult time with you. If your feelings are getting too much for you don't be afraid to talk to your doctor who can offer professional advice.

Sense of Loss

'I'll never be the same again'. 'I'm not a whole woman because I can't have children'.

These feelings are very understandable, especially if you are young and had been hoping to have children or to add to your family. Give yourself time to mourn this loss and talk it through with your partner or a close friend. It is, after all, very similar to a bereavement.

Learning to Cope

Women with cancer of the ovary have a lot to cope with — as well as the physical effects of their illness they also have to face the emotional consequences. In addition to all the other feelings we have talked about, you may also be worried that you will be rejected by your partner. If you can summon up the courage to talk openly about these fears you will probably find that they are unfounded. Intimate relationships are built on so many things — love, trust, common experience and lots of other feelings. You may even find new closeness in the relationship after working through the problem together.

Don't hesitate to seek professional help if you are finding the situation too overwhelming. Talking about your feelings can often help to clarify your own thoughts and give others the opportunity to understand how you are feeling. You may find it helpful to talk to someone who has been through a similar experience. BACUP has information about counsellors or support groups in your area.

Don't see it as a sign of failure that you have not been able to cope on your own. Once people understand how you are feeling they can be more supportive.

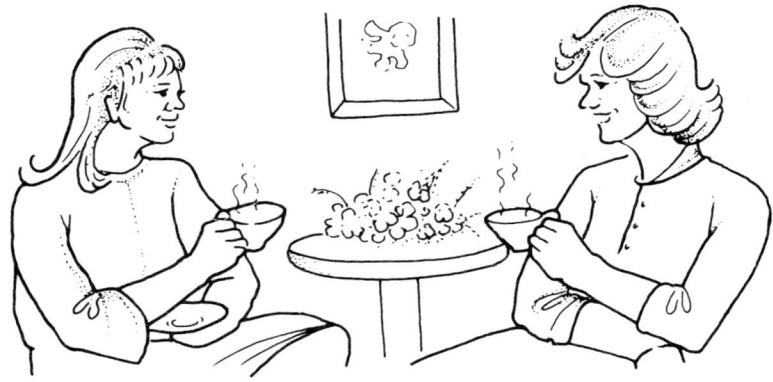

Who and What to Tell

Some families find it difficult to talk about cancer or share their feelings. The first reaction of many relatives is that the patient should not be told she has cancer. They may be afraid that she will be unable to cope with the news. If a decision is made not to tell the patient the family then has to cover up and hide information. These secrets within a family can be very difficult to keep and they can isolate the patient. They make her more frightened than she needs to be and they can cause tension between family members. In any case, many people suspect their diagnosis, even if they are not actually told.

Whether you are the patient or a close relative look out for friends and relatives with a positive attitude as they are always more helpful than the gloomy, pessimistic ones.

Relatives and friends can help by listening carefully to what, and how much the patient wants to say. Don't rush people into talking about their illness. Often it is enough just to listen to the patient and let them talk when they are ready.

Talking to Children

Deciding what to tell children about cancer is difficult. How much you tell them will probably depend on their age and how grown up they are. Very young children are concerned with immediate events. They don't understand illness and need only simple explanations of why their mother or friend has had to go into hospital. Slightly older children may understand a story explanation in terms of 'good cells and bad cells' but all young children need to be repeatedly reassured that the illness is not their fault. By the age of ten most children can grasp fairly complicated explanations.

Adolescent children may find it particularly difficult to cope with the situation because they feel they are being forced back into the family just as they were beginning to break free and gain their independence. Daughters in particular may worry that their mother's illness can be passed on to them.

An open honest approach is usually the best way for all children. Listen to their fears and be aware of any changes in their behaviour. This may be their way of expressing their feelings. It may be better to start by giving only small amounts of information and gradually building up a picture of the illness. But don't keep them in the dark about what is going on. Their fears are likely to be much worse than reality.

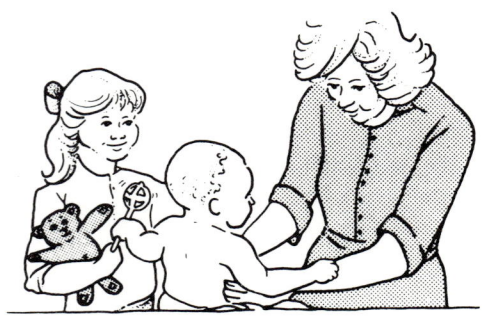

What You Can Do

A lot of people feel helpless when they are first told they have cancer and think there is nothing they can do, other than hand themselves over to doctors and hospitals. This is not so. There are many things you, and your family, can do at this time.

Practical and Positive Tasks

At times you may not be able to do things you used to take for granted. But as you begin to feel better you can set yourself some simple goals and gradually build up your confidence. Take things slowly and one step at a time.

Many people talk about 'fighting their illness'. This is a healthy response and it can be done by becoming involved in your illness. One easy way of doing this is by planning a healthy, well-balanced diet. Another way is to learn relaxation techniques which you can practise at home with tapes. Contact BACUP for more information.

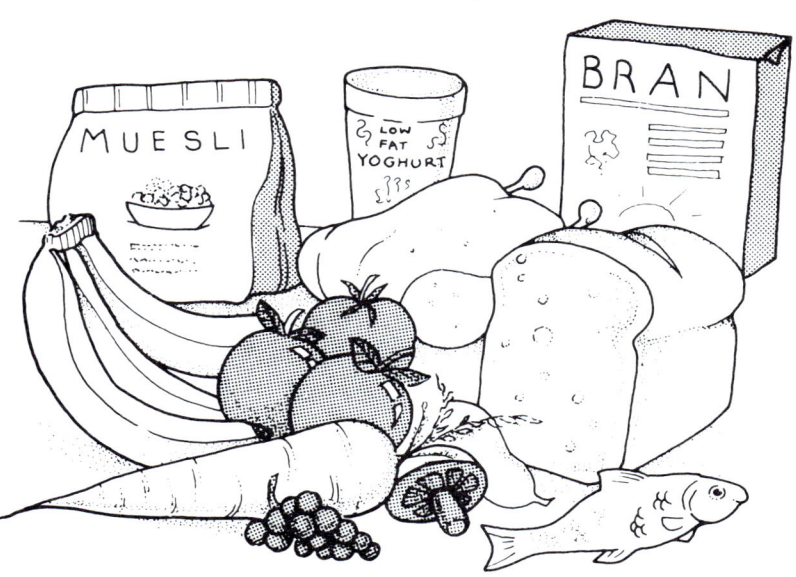

Many women find it valuable to take some regular exercise. The type of exercise you take, and how strenuous depends on what you are used to and how well you feel. Set yourself realistic aims and build up slowly.

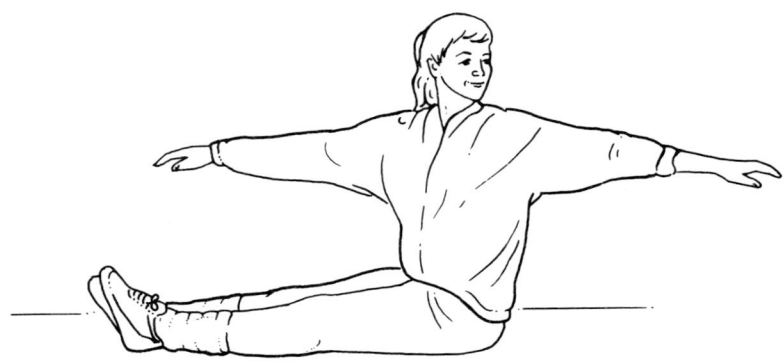

Understanding Your Illness

If you and your family understand your illness and its treatment you will be better prepared to cope with the situation. In this way you at least have some idea of what you are facing.

However, for information to be of value it must come from a reliable source to prevent it causing unnecessary fears. Personal medical information should come from your own doctor who is familiar with your medical background. As mentioned earlier it can be useful to make a list of questions before your visit or take a friend or relative with you to remind you of things you want to know but can forget so easily. Other sources of information are given at the end of this booklet.

Who Can Help?

The most important thing to remember is that there are people available to help you and your family. Often it is easier to talk to someone who is not directly involved with your illness. You may find it helpful to talk to a counsellor, who is specially trained to offer advice about various problems. Some people also find great comfort in their religion at this time. The nurses at BACUP are always happy to discuss any problems and they can put you in touch with a counsellor who lives near you or a local cancer support group.

There are several people who can offer support in the community. District nurses work closely with GPs and make regular visits to patients and their families at home. In many areas of the country there are also Macmillan and Marie Curie nurses, who are specially trained to look after people with cancer in their own homes. Let your GP know if you are having any problems at home so that proper home care can be arranged.

On the practical side it is worth checking up on the benefits and social services you can claim while you are ill. Social workers attached to the hospital or your family doctor can help you find out about these. For example, you may be entitled to meals on wheels, a home help or hospital fares.

For full advice on available benefits you can also contact your local Department of Health and Social Security (DHSS), the Citizens Advice Bureau or your local Social Services office. You can find the address and 'phone number of your nearest DHSS in the 'phone book under Health and Social Security. Social Services offices are listed under individual boroughs.

Sick Pay and Benefits

If you are employed, and unable to work, your employer will pay your first twenty-eight weeks sick pay. If, after this period, you are still unable to work you can claim Sickness Benefit from the DHSS.

If you are unemployed and not fit to work you will need to switch from Unemployment Benefit to Sickness Benefit. To do this you should contact your local DHSS office and arrange to send them regular sickness certificates from your doctor.

If you are ill and not at work do remember to ask your family doctor for a medical certificate to cover the period of your illness. If you are in hospital ask the doctor or nurse for a certificate, which you will need to claim benefit.

If, because of your illness, your income is 'less than your requirements' you may be entitled to Supplementary Benefit.

As these benefits are changing all the time it is advisable to contact your local DHSS office for up-to-date information.

BACUP's Cancer Information Service

This has been set up to give you and your family information on all aspects of cancer and its treatment, as well as on the practical and emotional problems of living with the illness. Information has been put together on computer about services available to cancer patients, treatment and research centres, cancer support groups, therapists and counsellors, financial assistance and home nursing services. Some of these are listed on the next few pages.

If you would like any other booklets, or help, you can 'phone us and speak to one of our experienced cancer nurses. Our Cancer Information Service is open to telephone enquiries from 10am to 5.30pm on weekdays, extended to 7pm on Tuesday and Thursdays. The number to call is 01 608 1661.

Other Useful Organisations

CancerLink
46 Pentonville Road
London N1
Tel: 01 833 2451

Resource centre for cancer self help and support groups throughout Britain and a telephone information service on all aspects of cancer.

Cancer Aftercare and Rehabilitation Society (CARE)
21 Zetland Road
Redland
Bristol BS6 7AH
Tel: 0272 427419

An organisation of cancer patients, relatives and friends who offer help and support. Branches throughout the country.

Cancer Relief
15-19 Britten Street
London SW3 3TY
Tel: 01 351 7811

Provides home care nurses through the Macmillan Service and financial grants for people with cancer and their families.

Hysterectomy Support Groups
c/o Ann Webb
11 Henryson Road
Brockley
London SE1 1WL
Tel: 01 690 5987 (Answerphone)

Offers information about hysterectomy and local hysterectomy support groups.

Marie Curie Memorial Foundation
28 Belgrave Square
London SW1X 8QG
Tel: 01 235 3325

Runs eleven nursing homes throughout the UK and a community nursing service to give extended care to patients at home.

Tak Tent
132 Hill Street
Glasgow
Tel: 041 332 3639

Provides training courses for people setting up groups. Produces written material.

Tenovus Cancer Information Centre
11 Whitchurch Road
Cardiff CF4 3JN
Tel: 0222 619846

Provides a counselling and information service personally or over the 'phone.

The Ulster Cancer Foundation
40-42 Eglantine Avenue
Belfast BT9 6DX
Tel: 0232 663281

Provides information over the 'phone about all aspects of cancer.

Recommended Reading List

Publications Available from BACUP

Chemotherapy
Radiotherapy
Diet and the Cancer Patient
Coping with Hair Loss

Publications Available from Libraries and Bookshops

Clyne, Rachael
Coping With Cancer: Making sense of it all;
Wellingborough, Thorsons Publishing Group, 1986

Dickson, A, Henriques, H
Women on Hysterectomy
Wellingborough, Thorsons Publishing Group, 1986

Haslett, S, Jennings, M
Hysterectomy and Vaginal Repair
booklet available from St Thomas Hospital, London, SE1 7EH

Smedley, H, Sikora, K, and Stepney, R
Cancer: What it is and how it is treated
Oxford, Basil Blackwell, 1986

'Which' guide
Understanding Cancer
London, Consumers Association Publishers, 1986

Williams, Chris and Sue
Cancer: A guide for patients and their families
Chichester, Wiley, 1986

Publications Available from BACUP

Diet and the Cancer Patient
Coping with Hair Loss
Chemotherapy
Radiotherapy
Cancer of the Bladder
Cancer of the Breast
Cancer of the Cervix
Cervical Smears
Cancer of the Colon and Rectum
Hodgkin's Disease
Cancer of the Kidney

Cancer of the Lung
Malignant Melanoma
Non-Hodgkin's Lymphoma
Cancer of the Oesophagus
Cancer of the Pancreas
Cancer of the Prostate
Cancer of the Skin
Cancer of the Stomach
Cancer of the Testes
Cancer of the Thyroid
Cancer of the Uterus

For further information please contact:

BACUP
121-123 Charterhouse Street,
London, EC1M 6AA

Cancer Information Service 01 608 1661
Administration 01 608 1785

BACUP's Cancer Information Service relies on voluntary contributions to maintain its services. We need your help. If you are interested in raising funds for BACUP, becoming a member or helping in any other way please contact us.

Typeset and printed in Great Britain by Lithoflow Ltd, London